PCOS

FERTILITY

COOKBOOK

SARAH JACK

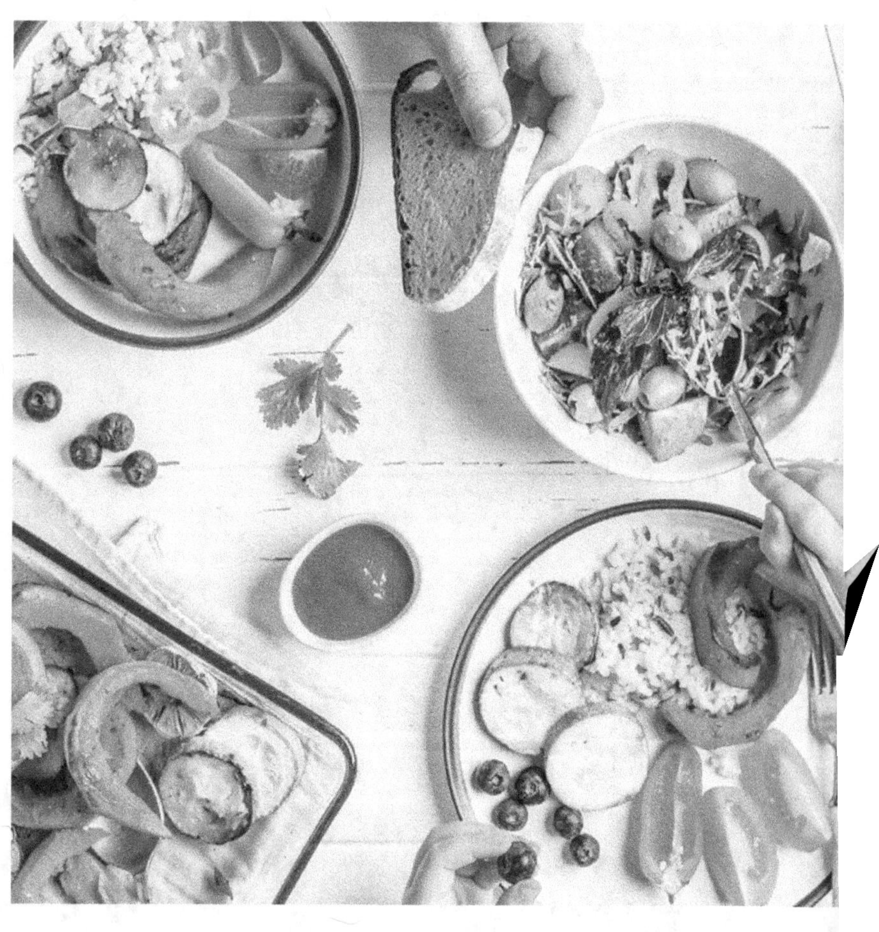

COPYRIGHT

3

All rights reserved. This book or any portion thereof may

not be reproduced or used in any manner whatsoever

without the express written permission of the publisher

except for the use of brief quotations in a book review.

TABLE OF CONTENTS

Table of Contents

COPYRIGHT 3

TABLE OF CONTENTS 4

INTRODUCTION 5

LIFESTYLE CHANGES FOR FERTILITY IMPROVEMENT 9

PCOS FERTILITY DIET 16

BENEFITS OF PCOS FERTILITY DIET 21

PCOS FERTILITY DIET RECIPES 26

INTRODUCTION

Some people with Polycystic Ovary Syndrome (PCOS) may encounter substantial fertility challenges, however it's vital to keep in mind that not everyone with PCOS will. People of reproductive age frequently experience PCOS, a hormonal condition that can cause irregular menstrual cycles, anovulation (lack of ovulation), and the growth of cysts on the ovaries. Some people with PCOS may find it more difficult to get pregnant as a result of these circumstances. Here are some important things to think about in relation to PCOS and fertility:

- Menstrual cycles that are irregular or infrequent are common in those who have PCOS. Because of this unpredictability, it may be challenging to estimate when ovulation will take place, which is essential for getting pregnant.

- Anovulation: PCOS can cause anovulation, in which the ovaries fail to release any or enough eggs. It is difficult to get pregnant without ovulation.

- Hormonal Imbalances: PCOS is frequently accompanied by hormonal issues, such as insulin resistance and high levels of androgens (male hormones). These imbalances have the potential to impair fertility and interfere with the reproductive system's normal operation.

- Lifestyle Factors: Hormonal abnormalities can be made worse by obesity, which is frequent in people with PCOS. In some situations, maintaining a healthy weight through diet and exercise might assist increase fertility.

- Medical Interventions: Lifestyle changes, ovulation-inducing drugs like clomiphene citrate, and assisted reproductive technologies (ART) like in vitro fertilization (IVF) may all be used as treatment options for PCOS-related fertility concerns. Based on your unique circumstances, your healthcare practitioner can assist in choosing the best course of therapy.

- Ovarian Cysts: One typical symptom of PCOS is the occurrence of ovarian cysts. These cysts are normally not the cause of infertility, but they can be a part of the overall syndrome.

- Emotional and Psychological Impact: Coping with fertility issues brought on by PCOS can be unpleasant on an emotional and psychological level. It's crucial to get counseling and emotional assistance when you need it.

If you are concerned about PCOS and its impact on your fertility, it's vital to talk with a healthcare provider, preferably a reproductive endocrinologist or fertility expert. They can assess your particular condition, carry out the required tests, and create a tailored treatment plan to assist you in achieving your fertility objectives. Additionally, treating PCOS and enhancing reproductive outcomes can be accomplished by maintaining a healthy lifestyle through nutrition, exercise, and

stress reduction.

LIFESTYLE CHANGES FOR FERTILITY IMPROVEMENT

Fertility is a complex aspect of human health, influenced by various factors such as genetics, age, and lifestyle. While some factors are beyond our control, lifestyle choices play a significant role in fertility. Making positive lifestyle changes can enhance reproductive health, increase the chances of conception, and contribute to a healthier pregnancy. In this comprehensive guide, we will explore various lifestyle changes that individuals and couples can incorporate to improve fertility.

- **Nutrition and Diet**

A well-balanced and nutritious diet is crucial for overall health, including reproductive health. Antioxidant-rich foods such as fruits and vegetables can help combat oxidative stress, which may negatively impact fertility. Essential nutrients like folic acid, zinc, and omega-3 fatty acids play a vital role in reproductive function. Additionally, maintaining a healthy body weight is essential, as both obesity and underweight can affect fertility.

- **Regular Exercise**

Engaging in regular physical activity is beneficial for fertility. Exercise helps maintain a healthy weight, improves blood circulation, and regulates hormonal balance. However, it's important to strike a balance, as excessive exercise, especially in women, can negatively impact reproductive health. Aim for moderate and consistent physical activity, such as brisk walking, yoga, or swimming, to promote overall well-being and fertility.

- **Manage Stress Levels**

Chronic stress can disrupt hormonal balance and negatively impact fertility. Incorporating stress management techniques such as meditation, deep breathing exercises, or yoga can help regulate stress hormones and create a more conducive environment for conception. Couples experiencing fertility challenges may also consider counseling or support groups to navigate the emotional aspects of the journey.

- **Adequate Sleep**

Quality sleep is essential for hormonal regulation and overall well-being. Irregular sleep patterns or insufficient sleep can disrupt the body's hormonal balance, affecting fertility. Aim for 7-9 hours of uninterrupted sleep each night to support reproductive health and optimize the body's natural rhythms.

- **Limit Alcohol and Caffeine Intake**

Excessive alcohol and caffeine consumption have been linked to fertility issues. It's advisable to limit alcohol intake and moderate caffeine consumption. Studies suggest that high levels of caffeine may interfere with the menstrual cycle and increase the time to conception. Choosing herbal teas or decaffeinated options can be a healthier alternative.

- **Quit Smoking**

Smoking is associated with reduced fertility in both men and women. It can lead to hormonal imbalances, decrease sperm quality, and increase the risk of miscarriage. Quitting smoking is a crucial step in enhancing reproductive health and improving the chances of a healthy pregnancy.

- **Maintain a Healthy Body Weight**

Both obesity and being underweight can adversely affect fertility. Achieving and maintaining a healthy body weight through a balanced diet and regular exercise is essential. Weight management is particularly crucial for women with polycystic ovary syndrome (PCOS), as excess weight can exacerbate symptoms and hinder fertility.

Stay Hydrated

Adequate hydration is essential for overall health, and it also plays a role in fertility. Water helps maintain optimal bodily functions, including hormone regulation and the production of cervical mucus, which is important for conception. Aim to drink at least 8 glasses of water a day, and more if you engage in physical activity.

- **Undergo Regular Health Check-ups**

Regular health check-ups are crucial for identifying and addressing any underlying health issues that may affect fertility. Conditions such as diabetes, thyroid disorders, and sexually transmitted infections (STIs) can impact reproductive health. Timely diagnosis and management of these conditions can improve fertility outcomes.

- **Educate Yourself and Seek Professional Advice**

Understanding the reproductive process and fertility basics is empowering. Couples trying to conceive should educate themselves about menstrual cycles, ovulation, and the fertile window. If conception doesn't occur after a reasonable period, seeking advice from a fertility specialist can provide valuable insights and guidance.

- **Conclusion**

Making positive lifestyle changes is a proactive and empowering approach to improving fertility. While there are no guarantees, adopting a healthy lifestyle can positively influence reproductive health, increase the likelihood of conception, and contribute to a healthier pregnancy. By incorporating these lifestyle changes, individuals and couples can take control of their well-being and enhance their fertility journey. Remember that every person is unique, and it's essential to consult with healthcare professionals for personalized advice tailored to specific needs and circumstances.

PCOS FERTILITY DIET

A healthy, balanced diet can be very important for managing PCOS and may even help with fertility. There is no one-size-fits-all PCOS fertility diet, but certain dietary choices and lifestyle modifications can support overall reproductive health by regulating hormones, enhancing insulin sensitivity, managing weight, and regulating hormones. Here are some dietary suggestions to take into account:

- Ensure that your consumption of carbohydrates, proteins, and good fats is balanced. Stay away from extreme diets and concentrate on consuming a range of nutrients from complete meals.

- Complex Carbohydrates: To assist regulate blood sugar levels, pick complex carbs with a low glycemic index (GI). Oats, quinoa, brown rice, legumes (beans, lentils), and non-starchy vegetables are some examples of whole grains.

- Lean Proteins: Include lean sources of protein in your meals, such as poultry, fish, tofu, lentils, and low-fat dairy. Blood sugar levels can be stabilized and appetites managed with protein.

- Include sources of healthy fats such as avocados, nuts, seeds, and olive oil in your diet. Omega-3 fatty acids, which are included in flaxseeds and fatty fish like salmon and mackerel, may have anti-inflammatory properties.

- Limit your use of added sugars, sugar-sweetened beverages, and highly processed meals. These might make insulin resistance worse and make you gain weight.

- Portion Control: Watch your portions to prevent overeating. If eaten in excess, even healthful meals can cause weight gain.

- Foods high in fiber can aid in satiety and blood sugar regulation. Increase your intake of fruits, veggies, and whole grains.

- Foods with Anti-Inflammatory Properties: Some foods may have anti-inflammatory qualities that can help PCOS. Turmeric, ginger, green tea, and foods high in antioxidants like berries are a few of these.

- Dairy Options: Some PCOS sufferers may benefit from selecting low-fat or dairy-free options because, in some situations, dairy products can impact hormone levels. Consult a dietitian or healthcare professional because this differs from person to person.

- Supplements: Discuss with your doctor whether you require any special supplements, like as inositol, which may occasionally aid with ovulation and insulin sensitivity.

- Keep yourself properly hydrated by consuming lots of water. Limit your intake of sugary drinks and too much coffee.

- Regular Meals: Strive to eat regular, wholesome meals on a daily basis. This may support regulating blood sugar levels all day long.

- Weight Management: People with PCOS who are overweight or obese can greatly increase their insulin sensitivity and reproductive results by shedding even a little amount of weight through a balanced diet and consistent exercise.

It's crucial to remember that people with PCOS may have different dietary requirements, and what works for one person may not work for another. In order to develop a customized food plan that is catered to your unique needs and goals, it is highly advised that you engage with a certified dietitian or nutritionist who specializes in PCOS. To make sure that your dietary decisions are in line with your entire PCOS management plan, including any recommended drugs or treatments, you should also speak with your healthcare physician.

BENEFITS OF PCOS FERTILITY DIET

When correctly planned and implemented, a PCOS fertility diet can provide various potential advantages for those with Polycystic Ovary Syndrome (PCOS) who want to enhance their fertility and general health. Here are a few potential advantages:

- Improved Hormone Balance: A PCOS fertility diet that is well-balanced can assist in controlling hormonal imbalances that are frequently linked to the condition, including as excessive levels of androgens (male hormones) and insulin resistance. Ovulation and menstrual periods may become more regular as a result of this improved hormonal balance.

- Enhanced Insulin Sensitivity: Insulin resistance is a common symptom of PCOS and can lead to weight gain and ovulation disruption. Complex carbs, fiber-rich meals, and stable blood sugar levels are all important components of a PCOS reproductive diet that might improve insulin sensitivity and possibly boost ovulation rates.

- Weight control: For people with PCOS, maintaining a healthy weight or losing weight when necessary, can help with fertility. An excellent PCOS fertility diet supports weight management through portion control and nutrient-dense foods.

- Increased Ovulation: Dietary adjustments can encourage regular ovulation in people who experience anovulation (lack of ovulation). A PCOS fertility diet may contain particular nutrients and supplements, including inositol and omega-3 fatty acids, to promote ovulation.

- Reduced Inflammation: Anti-inflammatory foods and spices like turmeric and ginger, which are frequently incorporated in a PCOS fertility diet, can aid in reducing the chronic inflammation connected to PCOS. Fertility may benefit from reducing inflammation levels.

- A nutrient-rich diet can assist the formation of healthier eggs, thereby enhancing the likelihood of a healthy pregnancy. Improved Egg Quality. Berries and other antioxidant-rich meals help shield eggs from oxidative damage.

- Better Emotional Wellness: Coping with PCOS and infertility can be emotionally difficult. A healthy diet helps improve mood and energy levels, assisting people in managing stress and the emotional ups and downs associated with infertility issues.

- Reduced Risk of Gestational Diabetes: By controlling insulin resistance with diet, people with PCOS may be at a lower risk of experiencing gestational diabetes, which is more common in PCOS-affected pregnant women.

- Healthy Pregnancy Outcomes: If you do decide to get pregnant, eating a balanced diet can help you have a healthier pregnancy by lowering your risk of developing conditions including gestational diabetes and preeclampsia.

- Adopting a PCOS reproductive diet frequently coexists with additional lifestyle modifications including consistent exercise, stress reduction, and sufficient sleep. These additional modifications can help to enhance fertility and general health.

It's important to keep in mind that while a PCOS fertility diet might provide a number of advantages, each individual may not experience the same level of success. Furthermore, not everyone with PCOS will have problems getting pregnant; some may need additional medical procedures or reproductive treatments. Working with medical professionals, such as a qualified dietitian or nutritionist, to create a custom PCOS fertility diet plan that suits your unique requirements and health objectives is highly advised. Additionally, seek advice from your medical provider to make sure that dietary modifications

fit in with your overall PCOS management strategy.

Cauliflower Fried Rice

Ingredients:

- 1 medium head of cauliflower, riced (or 4 cups store-bought cauliflower rice)

- 2 cups mixed vegetables (e.g., peas, carrots, bell peppers), diced

- 1 cup cooked and diced chicken breast (optional)

- 2 cloves garlic, minced

- 2 tablespoons olive oil

- 2 tablespoons low-sodium soy sauce or tamari

- 1 teaspoon sesame oil

- 2 green onions, sliced

- Salt and pepper to taste

- Sliced almonds for garnish (optional)

Instructions:

- If not using store-bought cauliflower rice, chop the cauliflower into florets and place them in a food processor. Pulse until the cauliflower resembles rice grains.

- Olive oil should be heated over medium-high heat in a sizable skillet or wok. Add diced mixed vegetables and minced garlic. The vegetables should be tender-crisp after around 5-7 minutes of sautéing.

- Stir in cauliflower rice and diced chicken breast (if usin g). Cook for a further 5-7 minutes while stirring continuously.

- Low-sodium soy sauce or tamari and sesame oil should be combined in a small bowl.

- Pour the sauce over the cauliflower fried rice and toss to coat evenly. Cook for another 2 minutes.

- If desired, garnish with thinly sliced almonds and green onions.

- Serve hot.

Baked Cod with Lemon and Herbs

Ingredients:

- 4 fillets of cod

- 2 finely sliced lemons

- 4 minced garlic cloves

- Olive oil, two tablespoons

- 1 tablespoon chopped fresh parsley

- 1 tablespoon finely sliced fresh dill

- Pepper and salt as desired

Instructions:

- Set the oven's temperature to 375°F (190°C).

- Cod fillets should be placed on a baking pan covered with parchment paper.

- Salt, pepper, and minced garlic are used to season cod fillets.

- Lemon slices should be spread over the cod fillets.

- Drizzle olive oil over the fish and lemon slices.

- Distribute evenly fresh dill and parsley on top.

- Bake for 15 to 20 minutes, or until the fish is flaky and well cooked, in a preheated oven.

- Serve hot.

Cucumber and Dill Greek Yogurt Salad

Ingredients:

- 2 cucumbers, thinly sliced

- 1 cup Greek yogurt or dairy-free yogurt

- 2 cloves garlic, minced

- 2 tablespoons fresh dill, chopped

- Juice of 1 lemon

- Pepper and salt as desired

Instructions:

- In a large bowl, combine thinly sliced cucumbers, Greek yogurt (or dairy-free yogurt), minced garlic, chopped fresh dill, lemon juice, salt, and pepper.

- Toss to coat the cucumbers evenly with the yogurt mixture.

- Refrigerate for at least 30 minutes before serving to allow the flavors to meld.

- Serve chilled.

Vegetables Roasted in Balsamic

Ingredients:

- 4 cups mixed vegetables (e.g., bell peppers, zucchini, carrots), diced

- 2 tablespoons balsamic vinegar

- 2 tablespoons olive oil

- 1 teaspoon dried thyme

- 1 teaspoon dried rosemary

- Pepper and salt as desired

Instructions:

- Set the oven's temperature to 425°F (220°C).

- In a large bowl, combine diced mixed vegetables.

- The marinade is prepared by combining balsamic vinegar, olive oil, dried thyme, dried rosemary, salt, and pepper in a small bowl.

- Pour the marinade over the vegetables and toss to coat them evenly.

- On a baking sheet, arrange the vegetables in a single layer.

- Vegetables should be roasted in a warm oven for 20 to 25 minutes, or until they are soft and have begun to caramelize.

- Serve hot.

Quinoa Salad from the Mediterranean

Ingredients:

- Quinoa, one cup

- 2 cups of veggie broth or water

- 1 cup diced cucumber

- 1 cup halved cherry tomatoes

- 1/2 cup red onion, finely chopped

- Pitted and sliced Kalamata olives, 1/4 cup

- 1/4 cup chopped fresh parsley

- Crumbled 1/4 cup feta cheese, if desired

- Extra-virgin olive oil, two tablespoons

- Red wine vinegar, 2 teaspoons

- 1 teaspoon dried oregano

- Pepper and salt as desired

Instructions:

- Quinoa should be well rinsed before cooking in water or vegetable broth per the directions on the package.

- Combine cooked quinoa, diced cucumber, chalved cherry tomatoes, finely chopped red onion, sliced Kalamata olives, and fresh parsley in a big bowl.

- The dressing is made by combining extra virgin olive oil, red wine vinegar, dried oregano, salt, and pepper in a small bowl.

- Drizzle the dressing over the quinoa mixture and toss to combine.

- Sprinkle crumbled feta cheese (if using) over the top before serving.

Lemon Garlic Shrimp and Broccoli

Ingredients:

- 1-pound large shrimp, peeled and deveined

- 4 cups broccoli florets

- 2 cloves garlic, minced

- 2 tablespoons olive oil

- Juice of 1 lemon

- 1 teaspoon lemon zest

- Salt and pepper to taste

- Chopped fresh parsley for garnish

Instructions:

- Broccoli florets should be blanched for two to three minutes in a big pot of boiling water. Drain, then set apart.

- Heat olive oil in a large skillet over medium-high heat. Add minced garlic and sauté for 1-2 minutes.

- Add shrimp to the skillet and cook for 2-3 minutes per side until pink and opaque.

- Add the steamed broccoli along with the salt, pepper, lemon zest, and juice. Cook for a further two minutes.

- Serve hot with freshly chopped parsley as a garnish.

Spinach and Feta Stuffed Chicken Breast

Ingredients:

- 4 skinless, boneless breasts of chicken

- Fresh spinach greens, 2 cups

- 1/2 cup feta cheese crumbles

- 2 minced garlic cloves

- Olive oil, two tablespoons

- 1 teaspoon dried oregano

- Pepper and salt as desired

- Toothpicks

Instructions:

- Set the oven's temperature to 375°F (190°C).

- Olive oil is heated over medium-high heat in a skillet. Add the minced garlic and cook for one to two minutes.

- Add fresh spinach leaves to the skillet and cook until wilted. Remove from heat.

- Wilted spinach and feta cheese are combined in a bowl. Add salt, pepper, and dried oregano as seasonings.

- Carefully slice a pocket into each chicken breast without cutting all the way through.

- Stuff each chicken breast with the spinach and feta mixture, then secure the pockets with toothpicks.

- Season the stuffed chicken breasts with additional salt, pepper, and olive oil.

- Place the chicken breasts on a baking sheet and bake in the preheated oven for 25-30 minutes or until the chicken is cooked through and no longer pink in the center.

- Remove toothpicks before serving.

Greek Chicken Salad

Ingredients:

- 2 boneless, skinless chicken breasts

- 4 cups mixed greens (e.g., spinach, romaine, arugula)

- 1 cucumber, sliced

- 1 cup cherry tomatoes, halved

- 1/2 cup Kalamata olives, pitted

- 1/4 cup red onion, thinly sliced

- 1/4 cup crumbled feta cheese

- 2 tablespoons extra-virgin olive oil

- 2 tablespoons red wine vinegar

- 1 teaspoon dried oregano

- Salt and pepper to taste

- Lemon wedges for serving

Instructions:

- Olive oil, dried oregano, salt, and pepper are used to season chicken breasts.

- Chicken breasts should be cooked through forabout 5-7 minutes on each side in a hot skillet over medium-high heat.

- Make the salad while the chicken is cooking. Combine mixed greens, diced cucumber, pitted Kalamata olives, halved cherry tomatoes, thinly sliced red onion, and crumbled feta cheese in a big bowl.

- Extra virgin olive oil, red wine vinegar, salt, and pepper are combined to produce the dressing in a small basin.

- Slice cooked chicken breasts and add them to the salad.

- Drizzle the dressing over the salad and toss to combine.

- Lemon wedges can be added to the dish for flavor.

Moroccan Chickpea and Vegetable Tagine

Ingredients:

- 1 can (15 oz) chickpeas, drained and rinsed

- 1 sweet potato, peeled and diced

- 1 zucchini, diced

- 1 red bell pepper, diced

- 1 onion, finely chopped

- 2 cloves garlic, minced

- 1 can (15 oz) diced tomatoes

- 2 tablespoons olive oil

- 1 teaspoon ground cumin

- 1 teaspoon ground coriander

- 1/2 teaspoon ground cinnamon

- Salt and pepper to taste

- Fresh cilantro leaves for garnish (optional)

- Cooked couscous or quinoa for serving

Instructions:

- Olive oil should be heated over medium-high heat in a sizable saucepan or tagine.

- Add the minced garlic and onion, and cook for two to three minutes.

- Add salt, pepper, ground cinnamon, ground coriander, and ground cumin. Cook for another 2 minutes.

- Sweet potato, zucchini, and diced red bell pepper arc added to the pot. The vegetables should be sautéed for 5 to 7 minutes until they begin to soften.

- Stir in drained and rinsed chickpeas and diced tomatoes.

- Simmer for 20 to 25 minutes, covered, or until the vegetables are soft.

- Serve the Moroccan chickpea and vegetable tagine over cooked couscous or quinoa.

- If desired, garnish with fresh cilantro leaves.

Spaghetti Squash with Turkey Bolognese Sauce

Ingredients:

- 1 spaghetti squash, halved and seeds removed

- 1-pound lean ground turkey

- 1 can (15 oz) crushed tomatoes

- 1 onion, finely chopped

- 2 cloves garlic, minced

- 1 teaspoon dried basil

- 1 teaspoon dried oregano

- Salt and pepper to taste

- Fresh basil leaves for garnish (optional)

Instructions:

- Set the oven's temperature to 375°F (190°C).

- Drizzle olive oil over the cut sides of the spaghetti squash and sprinkle with salt and pepper.

- Place the squash halves, cut side down, on a baking sheet.

- Roast for 35 to 40 minutes in a preheated oven, or until the flesh of the squash is easily shreddable with a fork.

- Cook lean ground turkey in a skillet until browned and well-cooked while the squash roasts. Drain any excess fat.

- Add chopped onion and minced garlic to the skillet and sauté for 2-3 minutes until softened.

- Stir in crushed tomatoes, dried basil, dried oregano, salt, and pepper. Simmer for about 10 minutes.

- Use a fork to scrape the flesh of the cooked spaghetti squash into spaghetti-like strands.

- Serve the turkey Bolognese sauce over the spaghetti squash.

- If desired, garnish with fresh basil leaves.

Thai-Inspired Quinoa Salad

Ingredients:

- 1 cup quinoa

- 2 cups water or vegetable broth

- 1 red bell pepper, diced

- 1 cucumber, diced

- 1 cup shredded carrots

- 1/4 cup fresh cilantro, chopped

- 1/4 cup peanuts, chopped

- 2 tablespoons sesame oil

- 2 tablespoons low-sodium soy sauce or tamari

- 1 tablespoon rice vinegar

- 1 teaspoon honey or maple syrup (optional)

- 1 teaspoon grated fresh ginger

- Juice of 1 lime

- Sriracha sauce for a kick (optional)

Instructions:

- Quinoa should be well rinsed before cooking in water or vegetable broth per the directions on the package.

- Cooked quinoa, diced red bell pepper, diced cucumber, shredded carrots, chopped fresh cilantro, and chopped peanuts should all be combined in a big bowl.

- In a separate bowl, whisk together sesame oil, low-sodium soy sauce or tamari, rice vinegar, honey (or maple syrup if desired), grated fresh ginger, lime juice, and Sriracha sauce if you like it spicy.

- Drizzle the dressing over the quinoa salad and toss to combine.

- Serve chilled.

Mediterranean Lentil Salad

Ingredients:

- 1 cup dried green or brown lentils, rinsed and drained

- 2 cups water or vegetable broth

- 1 cucumber, diced

- 1 cup cherry tomatoes, halved

- 1/2 cup red onion, finely chopped

- 1/4 cup Kalamata olives, pitted and sliced

- 1/4 cup crumbled feta cheese

- 2 tablespoons extra-virgin olive oil

- 2 tablespoons red wine vinegar

- 1 teaspoon dried oregano

- Salt and pepper to taste

Instructions:

- Dried lentils and water or vegetable broth should be combined in a saucepan. Bring to a boil, then reduce heat to a simmer. Cook for 20-25 minutes or until lentils are tender but not mushy. Drain any excess liquid.

- Cooked lentils, diced cucumber, cherry tomatoes, finely chopped red onion, sliced Kalamata olives, and crumbled feta cheese should all be combined in a big bowl.

- The dressing is made by combining extra virgin olive oil, red wine vinegar, dried oregano, salt, and pepper in a small bowl.

- Drizzle the dressing over the lentil salad and toss to combine.

- Serve chilled.

Lemon Garlic Shrimp and Asparagus

Ingredients:

- 1 pound of large shrimp, peeled and deveined

- 1 bunch asparagus, trimmed and cut into 2-inch pieces

- 4 cloves garlic, minced

- 2 tablespoons olive oil

- Juice of 2 lemons

- 1 teaspoon lemon zest

- Salt and pepper to taste

- Fresh parsley for garnish (optional)

- Cooked brown rice or quinoa for serving

Instructions:

49

- In a large skillet, heat olive oil over medium-high heat. Add the minced garlic and cook for one to two minutes.

- Add asparagus pieces to the skillet and cook for 3-4 minutes until they start to become tender.

- Peeled and deveined shrimp should be added to the skillet and cooked for two to three minutes on each side, or until pink and opaque.

- Add salt, pepper, lemon juice, and lemon zest. Cook for a further two minutes.

- If desired, garnish with fresh parsley.

- Serve with cooked quinoa or brown rice.

Veggie-Packed Egg Muffins

Ingredients:

- 8 large eggs

- 1 cup mixed vegetables (e.g., bell peppers, spinach, onions), finely chopped

- 1/2 cup shredded cheddar cheese (optional)

- Salt and pepper to taste

- Cooking spray

Instructions:

- Set the oven's temperature to 350°F (175°C).

- In a bowl, beat the eggs thoroughly.

- Stir in the finely chopped mixed vegetables and shredded cheddar cheese (if using).

- Add salt and pepper to taste.

- Grease a muffin tin with cooking spray.

- Each muffin cup should get an even layer of the egg mixture, about 3/4 full.

- Bake the egg muffins in the preheated oven for 20 to 25 minutes, or until they are set and have a light golden-brown top.

- Allow them to cool slightly before removing from the muffin tin.

- Serve as a quick and healthy breakfast or snack.

Turkey and Vegetable Stir-Fry

Ingredients:

- 1 pound of lean turkey meat

- 2 cups broccoli florets

- Snow peas, 1 cup

- 1 cup thinly chopped bell peppers

- 1 cup julienned carrots

- 2 minced garlic cloves

- 2 tablespoons of tamari or low-sodium soy sauce

- Olive oil, 1 tbsp

- 1 teaspoon finely chopped ginger

- 1/4 teaspoon crushed red pepper flakes (optional)

- Cooked brown rice for serving

Instructions:

- In a sizable skillet or wok, heat the olive oil over medium-high heat.

- Add the ground turkey and simmer, crumbling the meat as it cooks, until it is browned and well cooked. Take the turkey out of the pan and set it aside.

- Add the minced garlic, ginger, and red pepper flakes (if using) to the same skillet. For 1-2 minutes, sauté.

- Add broccoli florets, snow peas, bell peppers, and julienned carrots to the skillet. Stir-fry for about 5-7 minutes until the vegetables are tender-crisp.

- Return the cooked turkey to the skillet and add low-sodium soy sauce or tamari. Cook for another 2 minutes, stirring to combine.

- Serve the stir-fry over cooked brown rice.

Roasted Vegetable and Chickpea Bowl

Ingredients:

- 1 can (15 oz) washed and drained chickpeas

- 2 cups broccoli florets

- 2 cups florets of cauliflower

- 1 sliced red bell pepper

- 1 small red onion, sliced

- Olive oil, two tablespoons

- 1 teaspoon of cumin, ground

- 1/2 teaspoon ground paprika

- One-half teaspoon of ground turmeric

- Pepper and salt as desired

- Cooked quinoa or brown rice for serving

Instructions:

- Set the oven's temperature to 425°F (220°C).

- Chickpeas, broccoli, cauliflower, red bell pepper, and red onion slices should all be combined in a sizable mixing dish.

- Olive oil should be drizzled over the veggies and chickpeas. Salt, pepper, ground cumin, ground paprika, and ground turmeric should all be uniformly distributed. Toss to evenly coat everything.

- On a baking sheet, distribute the vegetables and chickpeas in a single layer.

- Vegetables should be roasted in a warm oven for 25 to 30 minutes, or until they are crisp and tender.

- Serve the roasted vegetables and chickpeas over cooked quinoa or brown rice.

Greek Salad with Grilled Shrimp

Ingredients:

- 1-pound large shrimp, peeled and deveined

- 2 cups cucumber, diced

- 2 cups cherry tomatoes, halved

- 1 cup red onion, thinly sliced

- 1/2 cup feta cheese, crumbled

- 1/4 cup Kalamata olives, pitted and sliced

- 1/4 cup fresh parsley, chopped

- 2 tablespoons extra-virgin olive oil

- 2 tablespoons red wine vinegar

- 1 teaspoon dried oregano

- Salt and pepper to taste

- Lemon wedges for serving

Instructions:

- A grill or grill pan should be preheated over medium-high heat.

- Olive oil, dried oregano, salt, and pepper are used to season shrimp. If desired, thread onto skewers.

- For about two to three minutes on each side, grill shrimp until pink and opaque.

- Cucumber, cherry tomatoes, red onion, feta cheese, Kalamata olives, and fresh parsley are all combined in a big bowl.

- In a small bowl, whisk together extra-virgin olive oil and red wine vinegar to make the dressing. Season with salt and pepper.

- Take shrimp off skewers, then incorporate them into the salad. Drizzle with dressing and toss to combine.

- Lemon wedges can be added to the dish for flavor.

Spinach and Mushroom Quiche

Ingredients:

- 1 pre-made whole wheat pie crust (store-bought or homemade)

- 4 large eggs

- 1 cup fresh spinach, chopped

- 1 cup mushrooms, sliced

- 1/2 cup red bell pepper, diced

- 1/2 cup onion, finely chopped

- 1/2 cup feta cheese, crumbled

- 1/2 cup milk (dairy or non-dairy)

- 1/2 teaspoon dried thyme

- Pepper and salt as desired

Instructions:

- Set the oven's temperature to 375°F (190°C).

- In a large bowl, whisk together eggs, milk, dried thyme, salt, and pepper.

- Combine the eggs, milk, dried thyme, salt, and pepper in a big bowl.

- Place the pie crust in a pie dish and spread the chopped spinach evenly on the bottom.

- On top of the spinach layer, put the sautéed vegetables.

- Pour the egg mixture over the vegetables.

- Sprinkle crumbled feta cheese evenly over the top.

- Bake for 35 to 40 minutes, or until the quiche is set and the top is golden, in the preheated oven.

- Allow it to cool slightly before slicing and serving.

Lemon Garlic Shrimp and Broccoli

Ingredients:

- 1-pound large shrimp, peeled and deveined

- 4 cups broccoli florets

- 2 cloves garlic, minced

- 2 tablespoons olive oil

- Juice of 1 lemon

- 1 teaspoon lemon zest

- Pepper and salt as desired

- Chopped fresh parsley for garnish

Instructions:

- Broccoli florets should be blanched for two to three minutes in a big pot of boiling water. Drain, then set apart.

- Over medium-high heat, warm up the olive oil in a big skillet. Add the minced garlic and cook for one to two minutes.

- Add shrimp to the skillet and cook for 2-3 minutes per side until pink and opaque.

- Stir in blanched broccoli, lemon juice, lemon zest, salt, and pepper. Cook for an additional 2 minutes.

- Serve hot with freshly chopped parsley as a garnish.

Spaghetti Squash with Pesto and Cherry Tomatoes

Ingredients:

- 1 spaghetti squash, halved and seeds removed

- 2 cups cherry tomatoes, halved

- 1/4 cup pesto sauce (store-bought or homemade)

- 2 tablespoons olive oil

- Salt and pepper to taste

- Fresh basil leaves for garnish (optional)

Instructions:

- Set the oven's temperature to 375°F (190°C).

- Drizzle olive oil over the cut sides of the spaghetti squash and sprinkle with salt and pepper.

- Place the squash halves, cut side down, on a baking sheet.

- Roast in the preheated oven for 35-40 minutes or until the squash flesh can be easily shredded with a fork.

- Use a fork to scrape the flesh of the cooked squash into spaghetti-like strands.

- Combine spaghetti squash strands, cherry tomatoes, and pesto sauce in a big skillet. Cook until thoroughly heated for 1-2 minutes.

- Garnish with fresh basil leaves if desired.

- Serve hot.

Black Bean and Sweet Potato Tacos

Ingredients:

- 2 medium sweet potatoes, peeled and diced

- 1 can (15 oz) black beans, drained and rinsed

- 1 cup red cabbage, thinly sliced

- 1/2 cup red onion, finely chopped

- 1/4 cup fresh cilantro, chopped

- 1/4 cup Greek yogurt or dairy-free yogurt

- 2 tablespoons lime juice

- 1 teaspoon ground cumin

- 1/2 teaspoon chili powder

- Salt and pepper to taste

- 8 small whole wheat or corn tortillas

Instructions:

- Set the oven's temperature to 425°F (220°C).

- Place diced sweet potatoes on a baking sheet. Drizzle with olive oil, sprinkle with ground cumin, chili powder, salt, and pepper. Toss to coat.

- Roast sweet potatoes in a preheated oven for 25 to 30 minutes, or until they are soft but still somewhat crunchy.

- Greek yogurt (or dairy-free yogurt) and lime juice are combined to create a creamy sauce in a small bowl.

- Warm the tortillas according to package instructions.

- Assemble the tacos by filling each tortilla with roasted sweet potatoes, black beans, thinly sliced red cabbage, finely chopped red onion, and chopped fresh cilantro.

- Add the creamy lime sauce in a drizzle.

- Serve the tacos warm.

Cucumber and Avocado Sushi Rolls

Ingredients:

- 2 cups sushi rice

- 4 sheets nori (seaweed) paper

- 1 avocado, thinly sliced

- 1 cucumber, thinly sliced

- 1/2 cup imitation crab sticks (optional)

- Soy sauce or tamari for dipping

- Pickled ginger and wasabi for serving (optional)

Instructions:

- Sushi rice should be prepared per the directions on the package and allowed to cool to room temperature.

- On a spotless surface, set a bamboo sushi rolling mat. The bamboo mat should be covered with a sheet of plastic wrap.

- One sheet of nori (seaweed) should be placed on the plastic wrap.

- Wet your hands with water to prevent sticking and spread a thin layer of sushi rice evenly over the nori, leaving about half an inch of nori at the top uncovered.

- Arrange avocado slices, cucumber slices, and imitation crab sticks (if using) on top of the rice.

- Carefully lift the bamboo mat and plastic wrap, rolling the nori and rice over the fillings to create a tight cylinder.

- Slice the sushi roll into bite-sized pieces using a sharp knife.

- With the remaining nori sheets and fillings, repeat the procedure.

- Serve the sushi rolls with soy sauce or tamari for dipping, and optionally, pickled ginger and wasabi.

Chicken and Vegetable Sheet Pan Dinner

Ingredients:

- 4 skinless, boneless breasts of chicken

- Broccoli florets, 4 cups

- 2 cups florets of cauliflower

- 1 sliced red bell pepper

- 1 sliced yellow bell pepper

- Olive oil, 1/4 cup

- 2 minced garlic cloves

- One tablespoon of dried thyme

- 1 teaspoon of rosemary, dry

- Pepper and salt as desired

- Lemon wedges for serving

Instructions:

- Set the oven's temperature to 425°F (220°C).

- On a baking sheet, arrange chicken breasts, broccoli, cauliflower, and sliced bell peppers.

- Olive oil, minced garlic, dried thyme, dried rosemary, salt, and pepper should all be combined in a small bowl.

- Drizzle the olive oil mixture over the chicken and vegetables.

- Toss to evenly coat everything.

- Roast for 25 to 30 minutes in a preheated oven, or until the chicken is cooked through and the vegetables are soft.

- Serve with lemon wedges for added flavor.

Greek Chicken and Quinoa Bowl

Ingredients:

- 4 skinless, boneless thighs of chicken

- Quinoa, one cup

- 2 cups of chicken broth or water

- 1 cup cherry tomatoes, halved

- Diced cucumber, half

- 1/4 cup red onion, finely chopped

- Pitted and sliced Kalamata olives, 1/4 cup

- Feta cheese crumbles, 1/4 cup (optional)

- Extra-virgin olive oil, two tablespoons

- Red wine vinegar, 2 teaspoons

- 1 teaspoon dried oregano

- Pepper and salt as desired

- Fresh parsley for garnish (optional)

Instructions:

71

- Salt, pepper, dried oregano, and olive oil are used to season chicken thighs.

- Chicken thighs should be cooked through after about 5-7 minutes on each side in a hot skillet over medium-high heat.

- Quinoa should be well rinsed before cooking, which should be done in the same amount of time as the chicken.

- Cooked quinoa, diced cucumber, finely chopped red onion, sliced Kalamata olives, and crumbled feta cheese (if using) should all be combined in a big dish.

- Extra virgin olive oil, red wine vinegar, salt, and pepper are combined to produce the dressing in a small basin.

- Chicken thighs are cut into slices and combined with the quinoa.

- Drizzle the dressing over the bowl and toss to combine.

- Garnish with fresh parsley if desired.

Sweet Potato and Chickpea Curry

Ingredients:

- 2 medium sweet potatoes, peeled and cubed

- 1 can (15 oz) chickpeas, drained and rinsed

- 1 onion, chopped

- 2 cloves garlic, minced

- 1 can (15 oz) diced tomatoes

- 1 can (13.5 oz) coconut milk

- 2 tablespoons olive oil

- 2 tablespoons curry powder

- 1 teaspoon ground turmeric

- Salt and pepper to taste

- Fresh cilantro for garnish (optional)

Instructions:

- Over medium heat, warm the olive oil in a sizable saucepan or skillet. Add the minced onion and garlic, and cook for two to three minutes.

- Stir in curry powder and ground turmeric and cook for another 1-2 minutes.

- Coconut milk, chickpeas, diced tomatoes, and sweet potatoes should be added. Add salt and pepper to taste.

- Bring to a simmer, cover, and cook for 20-25 minutes, or until sweet potatoes are tender.

- Serve the curry hot, garnished with fresh cilantro if desired, over cooked quinoa or brown rice.

THANKS   FOR

READING

THIS BOOK.

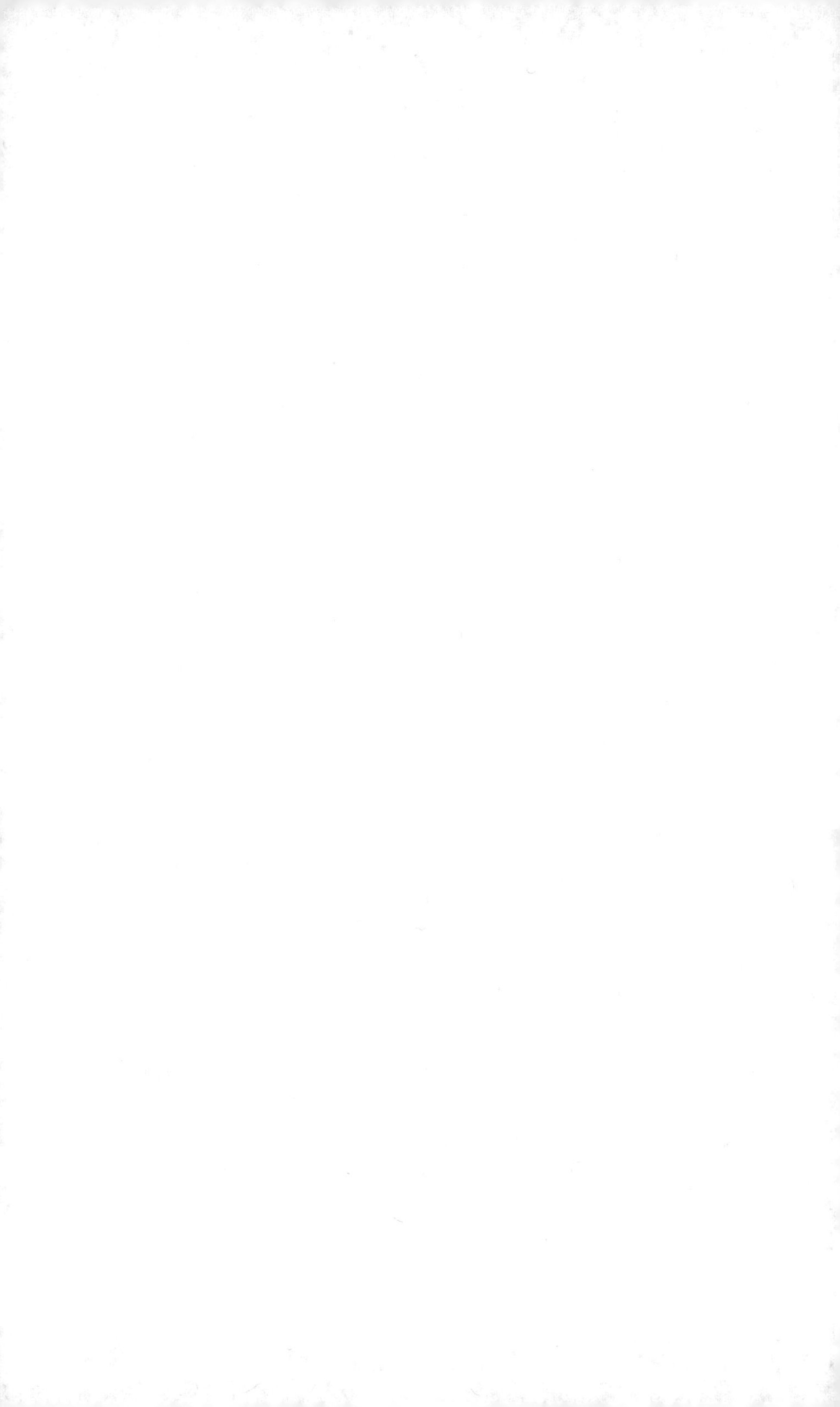